THE REMEDIAL USES OF HYPNOTISM

AN ESSAY

First Edition 1892
Frederic Gerrish M.D.

New Edition 2019
Edited by Tarl Warwick

COPYRIGHT AND DISCLAIMER

FOREWORD

This little pamphlet (for that is originally what it was) is a brief primer on the use of hypnotism within a medical setting, especially with regards to various "morbid" conditions such as overeating. Hypnotism is now generally regarded with less overall applause in the medical field and is relegated to a sideshow within psychiatry and as a vaguely interesting but not particularly useful facet of alternative medicine.

This is perhaps unfair. The placebo effect caused by suggestion has relevance within the subjective framework of the minds of those subjected to it; the only main issue with this present booklet is its considerably exaggerated account of the proportion of individuals able to be hypnotized- here it is above ninety percent, while reasonable expectations tend to be considerably lower, down closer to ten or twenty.

This edition of "Remedial Uses of Hypnotism" has been carefully edited for format and content. Care has been taken to retain all original intent and meaning.

THE REMEDIAL USES OF HYPNOTISM

The author expressly wishes it understood that, in issuing this article in pamphlet form, he is not in the least actuated by a desire to enlarge his practice in the neurological line, his special taste lying in an altogether different direction. Having found himself apparently alone among his immediate associates in his appreciation of the therapeutic value of hypnotism, he has endeavored in the past year to interest his fellow practitioners in this little-understood remedy, and this paper is one of the means adopted for that purpose. As, however, the transactions of the Maine Medical Association, to which the article was contributed, will reach only a part of the friends to whom he wishes to communicate his views and report his observations, he has had the essay put into its present form in the hope that the profession will more generally be persuaded to examine the subject in a judicial spirit, and afford the community the advantages to be derived from a proper application of hypnotic suggestion.

THE REMEDIAL USES OF HYPNOTISM

"Sunt verba et voces, quibus hunc lenire dolorem
Possis, et magnam morbi deponere partem."

The purpose of this paper is to awaken interest in an agency which has great therapeutic value, but is little appreciated by the medical profession of this State. The proper limits of such an essay are too narrow to permit a historical sketch of hypnotism, a presentation of its philosophy, or an attempt at explanation of its relations to various departments of psychical science. Suffice it, then, to remark on these intensely interesting and important subjects that the phenomena of what we now call hypnotism have been recognized, under one or another name, for thousands of years- in the present century quite commonly as animal magnetism, odylic force, mesmerism, electro-biology, neuro-hypnotism, and braidism; that the results of its application are attained probably through the channel of the imagination; and that the key to some of the most perplexing problems in psychology will possibly be found in this mysterious agency.

Hypnotism is an induced condition in which the mind is peculiarly susceptible to suggestion. (Suggestion is only the artifice employed to induce the phenomena. The real psychic mechanism of the process is still undetermined.) In our ordinary mental state there is a tendency to the expression of every thought in action- a tendency which long training has taught us to repress in the vast majority of instances. In the hypnotic condition thoughts which are presented are entertained with more hospitality, and are converted into actions in far greater proportion. As the etymology of the word implies, hypnotism is closely allied to ordinary sleep. Almost everybody is to some degree amenable to its influence, the susceptibility varying from nothing up to that state in which the person accepts suggestion

5

with hardly any obvious variation from his normal.

The number of people who are able to hypnotize others is much larger than is generally supposed. Probably any man who has those personal attributes which are essential to success in medical practice can affect his patients sufficiently to afford them the therapeutic advantages of hypnotism. Its employment is to be regarded, in general, as dependent not largely on a peculiar endowment of the individual applying it, but rather on a capacity in the person who receives it. And yet, while almost all of us can use it, the results obtained by some will naturally surpass those reached by others. The strong, reliant, imperious character is an element of success in this as in every other matter.

Belief in and knowledge of the practice, confidence in himself, a calm and equable demeanor, and abundant patience-these are the qualities which are requisite in the hypnotizer. On the part of the patient are needed a willingness to be hypnotized, and obedience to the directions of the physician. The patient's faith in the method is not a necessary factor of success; often brilliant results are achieved in cases where the patient is absolutely skeptical, and even jeers at the whole proceeding. Hypnotism is not a panacea; the claim that it is so comes only from the ignorant or the unscrupulous. But it is, in certain diseases, one of the most valuable remedies of which we have any knowledge. While it is possible that it may accomplish much in various other directions, it is highly probable that its chief victories will be won in the field of functional affections of the nervous system.

The hypnotic condition can be induced by various methods. That which I generally pursue is the following: The patient lying in a comfortable position on a couch, I close his eyes, and keep them shut by light pressure upon the edge of the lids. By gently spoken suggestions I encourage the idea that he is going to sleep, finishing with the assertion that he has gone to sleep. The process occupies a minute or less. The degree of hypnotization can be determined only by the application of tests. The patient, being in the hypnotic state, is ready for such suggestions as his case demands. These are made audibly, though the spoken word is by no means necessary if one can convey his idea to the patient by any other channel. I have repeatedly hypnotized and successfully treated patients without speaking a word, but my meaning was conveyed through the sense of touch.

In making the therapeutic suggestions, it is generally desirable to emphasize them by contact with the affected part. In some cases it is sufficient to do this through the clothing; but often this method fails, and the treatment does not succeed until the hand of the physician touches the integument covering the suffering organ. In almost any case the result is expedited by this contact. After the suggestions have been made, it is well to let the patient lie for a few minutes. Then he is roused by a word, which it is not necessary to speak loudly, for the hearing is rendered intensely acute during the continuance of the hypnotic condition. The patient must not be left until he is thoroughly awake. The hypnotic state is not of itself curative; the patient is put into it in order to receive certain suggestions, and after these have been introduced and allowed for a short time to impress the mind there is no object in continuing the hypnotism.

In a small proportion of apparently suitable cases the treatment is unavailing, even though the patient seems to be hypnotized. But as Prospero's brother says to Sebastian:

"For all the rest,
They'll take suggestion as a cat laps milk."

Of the cases in which I have had a fair opportunity, the hypnotic condition has been induced in ninety-five per cent. The greater part of these yielded at the first session; the remainder required two or three trials. If no effect was produced after three attempts, they were accounted unsuccessful. By fair opportunity I mean three sessions, if needed, and the cooperation of the patient. Only about one hypnotized patient in forty in my observation has been rendered unconscious, and yet in only three per cent, of them was there failure to get some remedial effect from suggestion. In ten per cent, the result was small; in twenty-five per cent, moderate relief was afforded; and in sixty-two per cent, very conspicuous benefit resulted. I use the expression "benefit resulted," because I have tested this treatment in so large a variety of cases, spread over so long a period of continuous work, and the relief, greater or less, has been so almost invariably the rule, that the question seems to me to have been clearly removed from the realm of coincidence. Chance will explain the phenomena in a dozen, a score, perhaps in several scores, of experiments ; but it will not give an adequate explanation to a rational mind in a thousand such trials.

Usually the beneficial effects of the treatment are immediately observed. The pain, which was agonizing ten minutes ago, has disappeared; the nervousness, which threatened an explosion of hysteria, has been replaced by a delicious calm; the depression of spirits and the feeling of unbearable fatigue are succeeded by cheerful placidity and a sense of refreshment. The effects are more enduring than those of any medicine which can produce similar results. As a rule the treatment must be repeated, sometimes daily, for a long time, but not as often or for as great a period as where drugs are depended upon. Best of all, in the opinion of some, is the fact that there are absolutely no unpleasant after-effects.

The nausea, malaise, head-heaviness, constipation, and anorexia, which are so likely to follow the administration of opium and other anodyne and soothing medicines, do not occur in consequence of a treatment with hypnotism. For more than a year past I have used hypnotism almost daily in my practice, and there is little in this paper which is not the result of my personal observation, which now covers about fifteen hundred applications. The report of a few illustrative cases which I am about to read must not be regarded as an adequate exemplification of the capabilities of hypnotic suggestion, since it includes nothing outside of the line of functional nervous diseases. Organic affections of the nervous system have but a languid interest for me, except when they have surgical bearings; and my practice has afforded no suitable opportunities to test the value of hypnotism in such cases, in which some observers have claimed grand results. For the production of surgical anesthesia hypnotism is not generally available, because so small a percentage of people can be put into the somnambulic stage, in which alone can operations of any considerable magnitude be performed without causing suffering. But a blunting of sensibility sufficiently pronounced to prevent pain in minor procedures, like the excavation and filling of carious cavities in teeth, can be accomplished with the patient in the lighter degrees of the hypnotic state, if the suggestion of freedom from pain be repeated incessantly during the operation. This fact I have not seen mentioned in any of the works on hypnotism, and I believe it to be a valuable discovery, the credit of which should be accorded to our fellow-member, Dr. Thomas Fillebrown, of Portland, Professor of Operative Dentistry in Harvard University.

At the risk of wearying by repetition, I will again mention the important fact that in almost all of my cases the patients have retained consciousness during the entire treatment, thus demonstrating the sufficiency of the lighter stages of hypnotism for the production of remedial effects. Some of the most striking results have been secured in the first stage, in which the patient can talk and laugh, and perhaps hardly feels at all drowsy. Of course, these slight hypnotizations fall far short of the requirements of the public exhibitor.

ILLUSTRATIVE CASES

The cases which I report are described with the purpose of illustrating certain prominent uses of suggestion, particularly in the production of sleep, the relief of pain, spasm, nervous dyspepsia, and tinnitus, the allaying of so-called nervousness, the correction of depraved appetite, and the dissipation of mental suffering. Hypnotism alone, and not associated with other remedies, was used in the treatment, in order that no question might be raised as to the agency producing the result. But it must not be inferred that hypnotism is incompatible with any other therapeutic means; it may be advantageously employed in connection with any other remedy.

Case 1: Insomnia.- A young married lady had been for a month subjected to great physical and emotional strain, incident to devoted attendance upon a near relative in a fatal illness. For three weeks she had had an average of not more than two hours' sleep in the twenty-four, and it had now become almost impossible for her to get any sleep. As was to be expected, she had marked distress in her head; and in addition she had a pelvic congestion, which occasioned much discomfort. One treatment with hypnotism dissipated all her troubles, and they did not return. For a number of days afterwards she slept refreshingly on every possible occasion. She required no further attendance for these ailments.

Case 2: Insomnia and Neuralgia.- A lady of past sixty had been a wretched sleeper for many years. Her nervous system was in a deplorable condition; she was in every respect feeble, and subject almost constantly to severe pain. In spite of treatment with medicines, electricity, massage, and the best of nursing, she was gradually drifting out of the reach of the usual remedies. I would not have been surprised at any day to find her stricken with paralysis, or killed by one of the frequent falls which her sudden attacks of weakness occasioned. At this stage hypnotism was tried, with immediate and gratifying effect. The neuralgia, which had resisted the largest doses of opiates which I dared to give, yielded at once; sleep at night became the rule, rather than the exception; digestion and nutrition improved, and her appearance was so altered for the better that her friends all commented on her healthier and happier countenance.

Occasionally, indeed, the old nerve-pain would return, but always to be routed after a short fight. This patient was somnambulized by hypnotism, and had no memory of what was said or done while she was in this condition.

She almost never slept in the daytime. One evening I put it into her mind that she would have an hour's nap, beginning at noon the next day. When the appointed time arrived she was overwhelmed with sleep, and did not wake for an hour. That evening I suggested, without her knowledge, that she should go to sleep the next day at eleven o'clock in the forenoon. At that time she happened to be out driving, and became so drowsy that only by strenuous efforts could she keep her eyes open and sit up in the carriage; and when she reached home she lay down and had the prescribed nap, which had been merely deferred by her exertions to keep awake.

Case 3: Spasmodic Asthma.- For a great many years a lady, aged seventy-two, had suffered from spasmodic asthma, the attacks lasting from one to three days, in spite of the assiduous use of the conventional remedies. Four times in the past year' hypnotism has been appealed to in these paroxysms, and has not failed to give perfect relief by cutting the attack short in a very few minutes.

THE REMEDIAL USES OF HYPNOTISM

Case 4: Epilepsy.- A girl of eighteen had for some years been troubled with petit mal, which was quite rapidly developing into the graver form of the disease. Almost every day there were some symptoms, the seizures generally being slight, but occasionally extremely disturbing, attended with marked confusion of mind and momentary unconsciousness. Immediate relief followed the employment of hypnotism; and the benefit has been so pronounced that there is the brightest prospect of complete cure. The case is still under treatment.

An almost identical case in a boy of the same age is receiving hypnotic suggestion, with similar effects.

Case 5: Neuralgia.- This patient, a lady of seventy three years, had been afflicted with neuralgia for fully half of her life. Drugs had never worked happily with her. On my return from a long vacation I found that she had been in distress for several weeks with the douloureux. She could not open her mouth to take food of any kind, or even to speak, without exciting a violent spasm of pain; and her sleep, never good, was greatly diminished in amount. On account of the insufficiency of her nourishment and rest she was plainly losing strength. Hypnotic suggestion immediately relieved her; but the pain returned again and again, so that many treatments were required. The attacks, however, steadily diminished in severity and frequency, her sleep was soon ample, and her ability to take food without pain increased rapidly. More than eight months have now passed since she has had an attack of tic, or of severe neuralgia in any part, and her sleep is thoroughly good- a satisfactory report of her condition such as she could not have made previously for many years.

Case 6: Neuralgia.- A carpenter, fifty-three years old, for a decade had had the douloureux, which had been so severe for two years past that his health was rapidly breaking down.

THE REMEDIAL USES OF HYPNOTISM

While giving his clinical history he was interrupted at every second or third sentence by a spasm of pain, which would relax after a few moments and permit him to proceed. Many a night was made utterly sleepless by suffering; and sometimes, when there would come a sudden remission of pain after a long-continued vigil, he has fallen to sleep on the instant at his bench with the implements of his trade in his hands. Commonly he could eat but two meals a day, and often only one, so greatly was the pain aggravated by the movements of the jaw. The usual, and some unusual, remedies had been tried faithfully but unavailingly; and he had come to depend upon morphine as the only thing which gave him comfort. Under hypnotic treatment he gained rapidly, and after the first application was able to eat three meals a day and to sleep all night. After twenty-three sessions he felt no need of further treatment for three and a half months, when the pain returned severely- only, however, to be routed in two days. I have not heard from him for five months, and infer that he has no need of further treatment.

Case 7: Neuralgia.- The patient was seventy years old and for more than half of her life had suffered almost constantly from neuralgia. She had long ago abandoned the search for relief, regarding it as fruitless; but, having observed the effects of hypnotic suggestion in a friend, concluded to give it a trial. The first few treatments produced hardly an appreciable result; but within a week she was so strikingly benefited that, in explanation of her sitting up for some hours beyond her wonted bedtime one night, she said that she wished to enjoy the sensation of perfect freedom from pain- an experience which she had not had previously for years- and, if she went to bed, sleep would make her unconscious of the novel blessing. Many applications were made at gradually increasing intervals, until weeks would elapse without need of treatment. It would be unreasonable to expect an absolute cure in such a case, so chronic and so unyielding to other remedies; but the improvement has been so great that the patient is vastly pleased with it, and is ardent in praise of the method by which it was achieved.

Case 8: Nervous Headache.- Every few weeks within her memory this patient, an unmarried lady of twenty-two years, had been stricken down for three and sometimes four days with violent headache. When I first saw her she was suffering severely with pain ; hypnotism relieved her in a few minutes. In a week she had another attack, and permitted it to get a strong hold before summoning me. My first attempt was only partially successful; but, after waiting a quarter of an hour, another trial was made, with perfect results. Thereafter, the headaches were far less frequent and less severe, the intervals became longer and longer until the habit yielded finally, and she is now apparently cured.

Case 9: Pain from Pregnancy.- In her two previous pregnancies this patient had suffered greatly from pain in the abdomen and back, and her physician had given her morphine daily, only partially relieving her distress, and seriously disturbing the nervous and alimentary systems. Though she was full of incredulity concerning hypnotism, four treatments by suggestion gave her complete comfort for three weeks; and afterwards an occasional application was sufficient to free her from all discomfort. This result is the more striking from the fact that the cause of the difficulty not only was not removed, but constantly increased until full term was reached and delivery occurred. The case is interesting also as showing that the patient's expectation or confidence in the method is not a necessary element of success in the practice of hypnotism. Patients often ask, "Must I believe in this in order to experience benefit?" And I always reply, "Certainly not. This is no faith-cure. You may be as skeptical as you choose." Their incredulity is of very little account- far less, in my opinion, in treatment by hypnotism than in that with drugs.

THE REMEDIAL USES OF HYPNOTISM

Case 10: Nervous Dyspepsia.- About twice in a year this patient, whose digestion has always been feeble, had an attack of dyspepsia, which usually kept her in bed for six weeks. Hypnotism, being tried on the last of these occasions, gave immediate relief, and in a week the patient had a good appetite, thorough and painless digestion, and was as near complete restoration as a month of treatment by ordinary means could bring her formerly.

Case 11: Nervousness.- A lady aged twenty-nine, an invalid for eight years, in whom the menopause had been artificially induced on account of ovarian disease, was a great sufferer from excessive irritability of the nervous system. She was in such a condition of tension that she seemed constantly to be in danger of a hysterical explosion. Pain was always present in the head, back, abdomen and breast, her sleep was scanty and unrestful, her mental state wretched, and she was continually taking bromides and other calmatives, occasionally even resorting to morphine. Hypnotism proved to be the only remedy capable of giving complete relief; and, while it has been necessary to employ it frequently, and doubtless it must be used for a long time to come, it has clearly demonstrated its vast superiority to all other means, and the patient is encouraged by the gradual but steady improvement in her health.

Case 12: Tinnitus Aurium.- Six months before consulting me this patient, a widow of fifty-five years, had an illness which left her with violent tinnitus. I do not remember whether or not she had been especially treated for it; at all events, it had increased rather than lessened after the lapse of a semester. Amelioration ensued at once upon hypnotic suggestion, and the cure was complete in five days.

Case 13: Morbid Appetite.- The peculiar character of this case may appeal to one's sense of the ludicrous; but nobody of ordinary good feeling could hear the patient's pathetic recital of her struggles, her defeats, and her constant misery without having his sympathy deeply drawn upon.

Hers was not one of the ordinary appetites, for the destruction of which the skill of the medical profession is so often invoked; but she had an insatiable craving for articles of food of an injurious kind- injurious, at any rate, when ingested in the enormous quantity which was habitual to her. She was wild for mince pie; the sight of ice cream and cake intoxicated her; confectionery excited a delirium of desire.

She would eat of such things egregiously, sinning all the time against light, but unable to control her actions. Every debauch was followed by a period of depression, in which she blamed and hated herself for yielding to the temptation, and yet, when next she was exposed to the allurements of bon-bons and pastry, of jam and jelly, they proved irresistible, and the former experience of unhappy delights and wretched dejection was repeated. She had made a confidant of nobody, and had borne this grievous burden alone for many years.

Being a woman of intelligence, education, independence, and sensibility, with high and noble ideals, her inability to keep above the pleasures of the table caused her to despise and and loathe herself so profoundly that she was in real danger of mental alienation. She received but a few applications of hypnotism, but proved to be an excellent subject for it, and consequently was immediately and powerfully influenced. She will probably need a somewhat prolonged series of treatments to effect a complete cure; but her letters are full of joyous descriptions of relief, and expressions of gratitude at her wonderful deliverance.

THE REMEDIAL USES OF HYPNOTISM

Case 14: Melancholia.- During a whole year this patient, whose age was sixty-nine, had been in a condition of melancholia. Her sleep was restless and insufficient, her mental condition deplorable. She was hopeless concerning relief, and absolutely incredulous as to the therapeutic virtues of hypnotism. However, being assured that lack of faith in the method would not affect the result, she consented to a trial of the proposed remedy, though she did not hesitate to pronounce it foolish. From the first night the sleep improved, and soon was abundant and refreshing. The depression of spirits yielded far less readily; but in a fortnight she was noticeably better, and in another month the cure was complete. The fretting, the fussing, the complaints about everything in herself and her environment, which were previously incessant, gave place to quiet good nature and cheerful interest in all that concerned her ; and, instead of being a nuisance to herself and a trial to her family, she became a normal member of society, taking enjoyment in the good things of life.

In most forms of insanity hypnotism appears not to be available. But in melancholia, where the power of concentration of thought is not lost, its influence may be great. Certainly, its value in this case is undeniable.

Case 15: Morbid Apprehension.- A lady, about thirty five years of age, who had been relieved of pain some months before by hypnotism, applied to me for help in a matter more serious than physical suffering. She said that she could not remember when she was not constantly haunted by the fear of assassination: some man was going to kill her with a knife. What put this idea into her head she could not conceive, but it was so firmly implanted that she was unable to get rid of it. She felt the necessity of keeping a light burning in her room all night, of having somebody in the house with her always. She sometimes would feel obliged to lock her chamber door in the day time, even though one of the servants was within easy call. Her husband's business often required him to be out late at night, and she never dared to go to bed until his return. Intellectually, she knew that there was no reason in her apprehension; but that knowledge did not give her the slightest comfort.

It is only fair to state that this patient is a woman of culture and refinement, of great sense and fortitude, and not at all hysterical. I have seen her get upon the table for a surgical operation with perfect steadiness. She is a lovely and judicious mother, and has the admiration and respect of a large circle of friends. She had never mentioned her trouble to any person before telling me of it. If she had come to me with this tale of a life-long horror before I had a practical knowledge of hypnotism, what could I have prescribed? No drug of which I have knowledge would have offered the smallest promise of relief. I could have told her to exercise her will to keep the hideous notion out of her mind; but what good would that have done when she had been trying that very thing for more than a quarter of a century.

She is very easily hypnotized, but never goes beyond the first stage- she can open her eyes and break the spell at any moment she chooses. I gave her a treatment of not more than five minutes' duration. In a fortnight she reported as follows: "I think the idea is in my mind about as much as ever, but I have no dread. If I wake at night and find the room in darkness, I do not get up and relight the lamp as I used to do, but immediately go to sleep again. I even go to bed in the dark- a thing which I never could do before. I never sit up for my husband now, but retire at the usual hour, and always sleep quietly. But I think that the fear is coining back a little." Three more treatments entirely eradicated the awful thought which had been the constant companion of her waking hours from her early childhood.

THE REMEDIAL USES OF HYPNOTISM

Though this report embraces cases of functional disease only, the seriousness of some of them is undeniable. I had grave fears for the life of one of these patients, and for the minds of several others. All of them, unless otherwise specified, had been in the care of reputable physicians, who had given them little or no relief. To my mind it is not always- perhaps not generally- the rapidly mortal cases which most reasonably excite our sympathy; but rather those in which the patients linger through years of irremediable suffering, longing for death but unable to die, a perpetual plague to themselves, and the occasion of unspeakable misery to others. For many of these wretched creatures the hopeless outlook of life is utterly changed by hypnotism. Cases which I formerly dreaded to visit, because of the impotence of my efforts even to palliate, become delightful on account of my ability to relieve. An addition has been made to my armamentarium which seems to me to deserve a place among the most precious of our remedial agents. I suppose that, if each one of us were to make out a list of medicines, and arrange them in the order of their usefulness, on a vast majority of the papers, opium, including its chief alkaloid, would be assigned the place of honor. Why? Because mainly of its anodyne properties. That certainly is the reason that the fathers of medicine called it *Donum Dei.* Our unanimity in according to it this prominent position in our materia medica is a sufficient evidence of the universality of physical distress, and of the character of much of the work which we are called upon to do. As has been often said, the medical profession would have a sufficient reason for existence if it did no other good than to relieve pain; and the drug which has been justly esteemed for ages as the principal analgesic still holds its place against all succedaneous medicines, though every year sees new claimants for the leadership. But I do not now use morphine as an anodyne in medical cases twice where I formerly exhibited it ten times, for the reason that hypnotic suggestion gives more prompt relief, is more enduring in its effects and leaves no unpleasant sequels.

THE REMEDIAL USES OF HYPNOTISM

OBJECTIONS ANSWERED

This paper would manifestly fail of its purpose if it did not answer certain questions which are prominently raised. Some of them are the outcome of prejudice; others are the product of ignorance, which has in some instances resulted from misdirected efforts at information. For instance, there are many physicians who, recognizing the great and trustworthy contributions of Charcot in other lines of neurological research, have adopted his conclusions concerning hypnotism, and have been most deeply impressed with his idea of the peril attending its use. But if they will observe that the experiments at the Saltpetriere, from which this conclusion was derived, were made upon a dozen hystero-epileptics for purposes of investigation and exhibition, they will have no difficulty in perceiving that inferences drawn from such data as to the nature of hypnotism and its effects upon healthy persons and in the cure of disease are extremely unlikely to be correct. The work of Charcot in this direction seems to me to have been inaccurate, and his deductions, consequently, misleading and unjust.

It is alleged that hypnotism is dangerous. The mind of the person who yields to its influence is said to be weakened by it. In answer to this I would call attention to the fact that hypnotism for exhibition purposes and hypnotism for therapeutic purposes are very different things. The one is harsh, often cruel, and possibly harmful; the other is gentle, helpful, and never injurious, if properly applied. The public displays of the phenomena of hypnotism by mountebanks are productive of no good (except to the pockets of the showmen), and should be condemned- the use of hypnotic suggestion by physicians for the benefit of suffering humanity is most commendable and worthy of every encouragement.

THE REMEDIAL USES OF HYPNOTISM

The only cases which I have seen reported in which hypnotism is justly chargeable with an injurious effect upon the mind, are those in which it has been employed for other than remedial purposes. Careful study of various works on the subject, and most scrupulous observation of the many cases in my own practice, seem to me to warrant the belief that no harm from hypnotism will come to the patient if the physician has such knowledge of the subject as is always presupposed in the employment of any remedial agent, and such discretion in its application as every member of the profession should possess. It would be as unwise and inexpedient to forbid all practice of hypnotism because it may be productive of harm in the hands of the ignorant, the reckless, and the unprincipled, as it would be to prohibit utterly the use of opium because the greater part of it is consumed in ways which are injurious to the race. Like many other valuable means which we constantly employ, hypnotism is not dangerous, if we bear in mind that it is dangerous.

In the second place, it is charged that a person who has been repeatedly hypnotized may become so susceptible to suggestion that he will easily fall a victim of vicious persons, to the great injury of himself and others. The possibility of this event is admitted- hideous crimes may have been committed by scoundrels who have made innocent somnambulists the instruments of their diabolical purposes. But if the use of hypnotism were to be restricted by law, as it is in Belgium, to members of the medical profession and other scientific students, this danger would be reduced to a minimum. The peril to society from this source does not appear to be great, certainly not at all commensurate with the benefits of the remedial application of hypnotism.

Furthermore, it is not difficult to protect our patients against this hazard through the agency of hypnotism itself. The patient may be locked by suggestion against hypnotization by anybody against his wish, and thus efficiently guarded against the danger which is apprehended. With the aid of Dr. Henry H. Hunt I have performed experiments which satisfy me on this point. A prominent physician whom I tried to interest in hypnotism said that it seemed to him "ridiculous," since it produced results only by influencing the mind of the patient. I confess to astonishment at this objection, as I had supposed that the profession, however divergent in belief on other matters, was united in considering it legitimate and desirable to help patients physically by producing an impression on their minds. Can it be that most of us have been doing a ridiculous thing these many years in trying to expedite recovery by cheering our patients, by inspiring them with hope, by cultivating their courage, by stimulating their wills? Is an agent to be denied admission to the ranks of remedies simply because it is psychic? Two evenings after hearing this objection I was called to a hysterical patient, whose condition closely resembled that observed in acute mania.

She was very violent, and had absolutely refused food for two days. Medicines had been administered in large doses. Treatment of the mind seemed to me preferable, but not with hypnotism. In her presence I expressed the opinion that, if she did not take food before midnight, it would be best to shave her scalp smooth. I had noticed that her hair was very luxuriant and well kept. Within thirty minutes of my departure she took a tumblerful of milk, with an egg beaten into it, and then immediately fell into a quiet slumber, which lasted twelve hours. This was the beginning of recovery, which thereafter steadily progressed. Now, I submit that this stimulation of the will was vastly better than giving drugs; indeed, I doubt if medication would have sufficed without the aid of mental treatment. I do not present this narration as an evidence of peculiar sagacity or of the smallest originality on my part. Many of you would have proceeded in a similar manner; and this method has doubtless been pursued ever since wise men began the practice of the healing art.

I report the case merely to illustrate my position, which is that the intentional employment of psychic means in therapeutics is often superior to the use of grosser agencies. If it is allowable to help the patient through the will, why is it not equally permissible to aid him honestly through the imagination? I am persuaded that the chief opposition to the use of hypnotism in medicine comes from ignorance of the subject, and that unprejudiced investigation will convince the profession that hypnotic suggestion is a mighty instrument for good.

It is not unlikely that some other physicians have the same idea of hypnotism as that expressed to me by an ex-president of this Association, who said that he considered it identical with "Christian science." I do not regard myself competent to judge of the appropriateness of the first part of the name of this epidemic delusion; the fitness or folly of the word "science" in its title may be seen if we consider the following statements, gathered from a somewhat careful examination of the subject as presented in its approved literature: First, a knowledge of anatomy and physiology is regarded not only as unnecessary, but even as positively pernicious. Second, the possession of physical attributes by objects in the natural world is due to the ascription of such qualities to these bodies by common consent; thus, if we all were to agree that aconite is a food and milk a poison, we would derive nourishment from the ingestion of the former, and would be killed by taking a drink of the latter. Third, the existence of disease of any kind or degree is absolutely denied. Of course, such stuff is pestilential rubbish; and it would be beneath notice in an essay on hypnotism, if crass ignorance of the latter had not led many physicians, as well as non-medical people, to confound the two. Hypnotism is not a religious fad; it encourages no fantastic conceptions of natural phenomena, it looks to the higher physiology for an explanation of its operations; it recognizes disease, and glories in being able to ameliorate the misery which disease causes, to attack it successfully sometimes in its citadel. No well-informed observer will assert the identity, or even close kinship, of hypnotism and the popular craze which masquerades under the misnomer of "Christian science."

But some physicians decline to look carefully into hypnotism, because they think (most unwarrantably) that it has always been in bad company. So said the Scribes and Pharisees of a certain one, whom they were incapable of appreciating. But, supposing the statement to be true, which it conspicuously is not, shall we leave this good thing, even though it has come out of the scientific Nazareth, to the publicans and sinners, the lepers and the harlots of medicine? Wesley was bright enough to see that the devil ought not to have all of the good tunes. We ought to be sufficiently sagacious to perceive that no good thing in medicine should be left to the monopoly pf the quacks. We should accept truth, whatever its source. Medicine has often profited by information derived from obscure, humble, and even disreputable quarters. The really wise man is perfectly willing to be taught by anybody who knows. In accepting hypnotism as a remedy, we do not need to take any of the grotesque garments in which charlatanry has arrayed it; we are not obliged to subscribe to the extravagant claims which over-enthusiasm has made for it. In the words of Flammarion: "Can we not find the happy medium between absolute negation and dangerous credulity? Is it reasonable either to deny everything which we do not comprehend, or to accept all the fantasies engendered in the vortex of disordered imaginations ? Can we not achieve at the same time the humility which becomes the weak and the dignity which befits the strong?"

THE END